MEDICA

FOR THE LAZY MAN

2019

SIMPLEST & EASIEST GUIDE EVER!

Copyright 2019 Douglas B. Jones, CLU, RHU

Douglas B. Jones, CEO, Associated Consultants of Arizona, LLC
DBJ@ACONAZ.COM

This book and the content herein have been written in order to educate and to simplify a complex subject. Every effort has been made to ensure the accuracy of the content, but there is always room for misunderstanding and misinterpretation. Therefore, no liability is assumed for losses or damages due to the information provided.

The reader is responsible for his own choices, actions and results. He should seek guidance from professionals whenever there is any question as to the advisability of a particular course of action.

WHAT READERS SAY:

Roy Brotherhood

Great how-to guide to Medicare!
August 30, 2018
Format: Paperback **Verified Purchase**

I am already on Medicare and did not need this book. I purchased it out of curiosity to see if it took the mystery and fear out of finding a good policy. I was pleasantly surprised to find how well it is written in simple terms and easy to understand.

Typically if you want to find out this information you have to submit your personal/contact information to an insurance company (or agent) and wait for them to call and put the pressure on you to purchase what they offer. This simple book eliminates that hassle completely. While the author offers to assist you, it is your choice to make the contact.

I recommend this book to anyone approaching Medicare age and if you are already on Medicare and want to change your policy this will be an excellent guide to do so.

Leigh Siegel
October 7 at 10:50 AM ·
Amazon

·

This is an incredible little book that will guide you through the Medicare process with ease and an incredible sense of humor. I feel so knowledgeable about the subject and I know exactly what I will do when the time comes to enroll.

Thank you Douglas B. Jones

Don't delay! Buy this book today and enjoy! I'm a GTO...
#greatread #medicare #Amazon

THIS BOOK IS DEDICATED TO:

<u>Lazy Men</u> too smart to waste time and energy on stupidity;

-PLUS-

<u>Lazy Ladies</u> who love them (...and who feel the same way!)

I am right there with you my brothers and sisters!

****

Do you live in:

Massachusetts, Minnesota, or Wisconsin?

If so, the information on **Medicare supplement plans** contained within this book will not apply to you.

Those three states have special Medicare supplement plans which are not marketed anywhere else in the United States.

However, the information on Medicare Parts A & B as well as information on Prescription Drug Plans (PDP) is accurate for you.

Coming soon.....

MEDICARE IN SECONDS.com

Purchase your Medicare Supplement
from me – ON LINE!

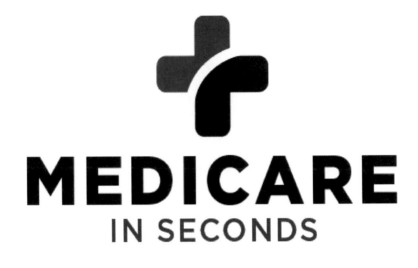

CONTACT ME:

DBJ@MedicareInSeconds.com

Would a GLOSSARY or FAQ be helpful?
www.MedicareInSeconds.com

My new website will seek to get you through the Medicare confusion quickly and painlessly with results that will serve you well for years to come. Maybe forever!

Within seconds your Medicare choices will be clarified and explained, but the confusing minutia and nonsensical details will be ignored (unless you want to learn more).

On MedicareInSeconds.com, you will find links for:

- Enrolling in Medicare Part A and Part B – from the comfort of your own computer.

- Finding the cost and buying your Medicare supplement plan to insure against financial loss due to the gaps and flaws in Medicare coverage.

- Easy steps to choosing the least expensive Prescription Drug Plan available in your area.

- All of the other exciting insurance information I could find to entertain and amuse!

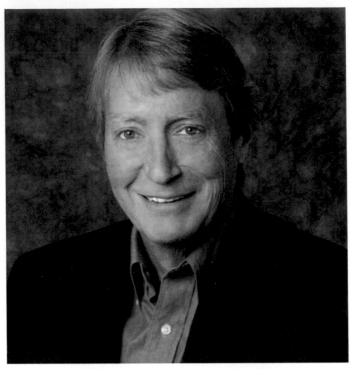

ABOUT THE AUTHOR

Douglas B. Jones, CLU, RHU

Medicare snuck up on me just as it does with most Americans.

As a long-time health insurance professional, I was expected by friends and clients to be ahead of the curve. Turns out I needed to educate myself on this complex subject in order to be able to offer solid advice.

After graduation from the University of Arizona I joined my family's John Hancock insurance agency in Chicago's Loop. Even though life insurance sales with the John Hancock was a 3-generation family calling, I found more satisfaction in helping clients with their medical insurance needs.

Eventually the company stopped offering those products, so I left to pursue my mission with other companies.

Decades later at a social event, I was asked by several people for a short version of my Medicare advice. They assumed I must be an expert since we were all rapidly approaching age 65.

That was the catalyst that convinced me to learn what Medicare was all about. After a period of study, I formed some conclusions that are directly at odds with other Medicare advisors.

One evening a couple of longtime friends came over to act as my Guinea pigs. The wife, ever the serious student, was lugging all of the printed material they had received and expected me to educate them on every one of the Medicare options available in our area.

The husband was mostly interested in the beer I offered. His opinion was that this whole Medicare decision process was an unpleasant inconvenience that should end quickly.

Within seconds, these friends had a complete grasp of my best Medicare advice and the reasons behind it. They were stunned that the whole thing could be boiled down to such a simple conclusion. As they discovered, the most time-consuming part of the process was completing the insurance paperwork.

That evening set the pattern for virtually all of my subsequent encounters with Medicare eligible citizens. Only recently did it occur to me that the same process could be offered to everyone in the country who was staring down the barrel of Medicare.

Thus, was born Medicare for the Lazy Man!

INTRODUCTION

How may I help you?

Nobody in their right mind would voluntarily read a book about Medicare (without a pretty good reason).

What's your excuse?

- Are you closing in on Medicare age?
- Considering leaving job-related insurance coverage?
- Responsible for advising a friend or relative?
- Reexamining the choices, you made years ago?
- Suffering from insomnia?
- Paying the price for a dissolute life?

Seeking a quick and painless guide through the Medicare maze?

LOOK NO FARTHER THAN CHAPTER 1!

What is the destination?

Until I dragged her out west to the University of Arizona, my wife attended a Catholic grade school and Jr. High, a Catholic girl's academy and a Catholic Women's college.

Eventually I realized that Catholic schools do not teach geography because she cannot navigate her way out of a wet paper bag.

However, after reading this very short road map and following my suggestions, you will have no problem selecting and acquiring the four essential layers of coverage necessary for complete protection under Medicare:

MEDICARE PART A

MEDICARE PART B

MEDICARE SUPPLEMENT PLANS

PRESCRIPTION DRUG PLANS

That is all you need for complete protection.

It is very likely that these coverages will serve you well for the many decades of life you have yet to enjoy.

There will be no need or requirement to do an annual review or renewal for anything except perhaps the Prescription Drug Plan and then only if you want to make sure your costs are reasonable.

The purpose of this book is simplification of a very complex subject and relief of the angst that many feel when the time comes to make decisions about Medicare coverage.

Among these pages the average citizen confronting Medicare for the first time will discover a short, direct path from start to finish that will relieve their concerns and possibly save them some money.

Notice I said, "average citizen".

The recommendations in this book are not for everyone, but the target audience includes the majority of those approaching Medicare eligibility.

Most helped will be people responsible for their own health insurance, specifically those about to turn 65 and those employed people contemplating retirement and termination from an employer's health insurance plan.

Those who are destitute and/or stricken with debilitating medical conditions should drop this book and seek advice from their state's Medicaid (welfare) office as well as insurance agents in their immediate locale. Most areas of the US have "special needs plans" locally available and designed specifically for people in dire straits.

Once again, **if you are infirm and/or destitute, stop reading right now and try to get a refund. This book is not for you!**

A NOTE ABOUT NOMENCLATURE

PARTS vs. PLANS

Original Medicare consists of two elements called **PARTS:**

PART A   PART B

Coverages that supplement Medicare are called **PLANS:**

MEDICARE SUPPLEMENT PLANS and **PRESCRIPTION DRUG PLANS (PDP)**

Two other elements of Medicare you will sometimes encounter are **PART C and PART D.** You should forget about them.

Part C plans are inferior; I do not recommend or sell them.

Part D is just another label for **Prescription Drug Plans or PDPs.**

<u>In this book I will only discuss:</u>

MEDICARE PART A

MEDICARE PART B

MEDICARE SUPPLEMENT PLANS

PRESCRIPTION DRUG PLANS

<u>THESE FOUR PROVIDE THE BEST PROTECTION AVAILABLE!</u>

Table of Contents

CHAPTER 1

Possibly the Only Part of This Book You Will Need!

Are you in charge of your own health insurance and hoping to simplify the Medicare coverage selection process?

The next few pages will allow you to ignore the prevailing confusion and purchase the best, most comprehensive medical insurance available.

STEP 1.

Have you selected your Medicare Part A start date?
(Read more in Chapter 3)

Have you selected your Medicare Part B start date?
(Read more in Chapter 4)

ENROLL IN MEDICARE ONLINE HERE:
https://www.ssa.gov/medicare/
The enrollment process could take as little as 10 minutes.

Only two more steps to go.

STEP 2.

Apply for your Medicare supplement plan to be effective on the same date as your Medicare Part B

CHOOSE YOUR MEDICARE SUPPLEMENT PLAN

These are the only two plans I recommend and sell:

High Deductible Plan F (HDF)	**Plan F**
High Performance GTO	Luxurious Cadillac Plan
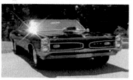	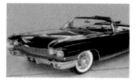
COST EFFECTIVE	**COMPREHENSIVE**
Lowest Monthly Cost	Moderately Higher Cost

HIGH DEDUCTIBLE PLAN F	vs	PLAN F
Recommended for people in these categories:		
HDF	**VS**	**PLAN F**
Average to good	**HEALTH**	All levels
Modest or better	**FINANCES**	Comfortable
Medium / High	**RISK TOLERANCE**	Low
Some out-of-pocket costs	**PERSONAL PREFERENCE**	No cost sharing
Low monthly premium	" "	100% Coverage

Premium Comparison	
Blue Cross / Blue Shield of Illinois 2018	
High Deductible Plan F (HDF)	**PLAN F**
Age 65: $48 / month	Age 65: $158 / month
Age 70: $62 / month	Age 70: $211 / month

Read more about Medicare supplement plans in Chapters 5, 6 & 7.

Only one more step to go!

STEP 3.

Select the least expensive Prescription Drug Plan (PDP)

from a list of all plans available in your ZIP code.

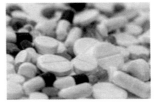

Purchase that plan online directly from the insurance company.

In **Chapter 9** you will find step-by-step navigation instructions leading you to that list of PDP plans arranged in order of annual cost.

These instructions look complicated, but it is a government website and so was not designed to be user-friendly. The most difficult part of the process will be entering the detail for each of your current prescription medications.

Since the PDPs are one-year contracts, annual costs can change at the discretion of each insurance company. Also, your prescription drug needs may change during the course of the year.

Therefore, you may find this a worthwhile project to do each year before the Annual Election Period (AEP) in the fall, in case you would like to buy a new plan for the following year.

If you were able to complete all three of these steps, you now have acquired the four essential elements of protection:

MEDICARE PART A

MEDICARE PART B

MEDICARE SUPPLEMENT PLAN

PRESCRIPTION DRUG PLAN

CHAPTER 2

What Does Medicare Do?

Illustrated by a fairy tale with roots in Chicago.

Medicare is a universal health insurance program provided primarily to Americans age 65+ by the federal government. It is intended to pay some of the cost of necessary medical treatment.

As an example, my favorite clients, the Sappertickers turned age 65 a while back and, with my guidance, signed up for Medicare through the government on its "oh so user-friendly" website.

Because they understood that Medicare coverage is full of gaps and flaws, they also purchased insurance to protect themselves from those weaknesses in the program - insurance to supplement Medicare known as a Medicare supplement. Clever, huh?

As luck would have it, Mr. & Mrs. Sapperticker have a cute little grandchild who spends part of every day in a bubbling germ factory known as nursery school. Upon receiving hugs from this grandchild, they contracted a major dose of the most contagious flu of the season.

Surviving this disease required several days in a hospital and some follow-up visits with the family doctor after being released from confinement.

Hooty Sapperticker expected massive medical bills to start arriving shortly after they recovered, but that did not happen.

The Sappertickers' medical bills, from the hospital, the doctors, the laboratory etc. were all sent to the federal government for payment.

This process started as the patients showed their ID cards to office staff when treatment began. Eventually those medical professionals all received checks for partial payment, again because Medicare coverage has many gaps and flaws.

Once the government (in the guise of Medicare) paid its portion, the providers turned to the Medicare supplement insurance purchased by their patients. They knew where to send their "balance bills" because the Sappertickers presented ID cards given to them when this supplementary insurance became effective.

Months after their full recovery, the financial consequences of their illness were resolved. The very conservative Mrs. Sapperticker had purchased the Cadillac of all Medicare supplement plans and paid a monthly premium of around $160.

She was delighted to find that her medical bills were paid in full – 100% coverage.

On the other hand, Hooty has always been more of a risk-taking party animal. He had purchased the Pontiac GTO of Medicare supplement plans for about $50 per month.

Hooty had to write checks for a few hundred dollars in cost sharing because of the deductible his plan carries, but this was more than offset by the $110 he saves each month in lower premiums. In addition, his beer funds have been protected from bill collectors.

The happy conclusion is that I, as the Sapperticker family insurance advisor, have been elevated to heroic status and toasted in absentia every time they gather together.

The cute little grandchild was never told about all of the misery caused by his grandparents' unconditional love.
SO, WHAT IS THE BIG DEAL ABOUT MEDICARE, ANYWAY?

Now that we understand Medicare is a simple bill paying mechanism for those Americans it covers, why is there such a hoo-rah about it?

Why are hapless citizens in their middle sixties accosted with piles of insurance company propaganda and endless warnings about the dangers of charging into Medicare without professional guidance?

All of this hysteria exists because of the Baby Boomers who are passing through middle age like a fat rat through a snake. As they enter Medicare (at the rate of 10,000 per day we are told) the market for Medicare supplement insurance has become huge.

Insurance sales people (known as leeches in some circles) are salivating uncontrollably at the income potential this population surge represents. However, they know how little you would need them if you hadn't been warned that their professional expertise was essential.

They desperately want you to trust them so that you will buy your supplementary insurance from them.
It is all about the commissions, folks!

Other, more altruistic advisors have intoned that responsible citizens must thoroughly read piles of insurance company propaganda, Medicare-related textbooks and other scholarly tomes.

They also suggest attending educational seminars and meeting with government officials in their offices.

 The implication is that you risk financial disaster and eternal damnation if you do not study and memorize all aspects of the Medicare morass.

This is a complete load!

Studying all of the minutia about Medicare is a huge waste of time and effort....unless you enjoy that sort of thing of course.

Why? Because knowledge does NOT equal power! Nothing you memorize about Medicare will allow you to improve it in order to get better or cheaper protection. Also, any implication that disaster will ensue if your Medicare selections are not absolutely perfect is equally false.

In reality, very few Medicare decisions are completely irrevocable; mistakes and poor choices can usually be fixed within a year or less. In fact, the most costly mistakes actually stem from refusal to act, as in the case of late enrollment penalties.

The good news is that, as stated in the Introduction above, among these pages the average citizen confronting Medicare for the first time will discover a short, direct path from start to finish that will relieve their concerns and perhaps save them some money.

My book has been written for those with:
Average or better financial resources
Average or better health
No desire to waste time or effort studying Medicare

Full disclosure department:

The reader should have realized by now that I also am an insurance salesman and "Medicare advisor". The reader should also be aware that I love commissions just as much as my fellow leeches.

However, my mission is one of simplification and relief of angst. An educated consumer should have no reason to fear the Medicare coverage selection process after reading my recommendations.

CHAPTER 3

Medicare Part A

Your goal in buying, borrowing or stealing this book should be to minimize the time and effort required to establish your Medicare related coverages. Let's get to it!

MEDICARE PART A is health insurance provided by the Federal government. It is intended to reimburse some expenses incurred during treatment in an inpatient facility (hospital, skilled nursing and rehabilitation).

In almost all cases, Americans with a 10-year work history (or those married to someone with a 10-year history of taxable employment) will have Part A provided to them free of charge.

Since it is free, almost everyone is advised to enroll in Part A coincident with their 65th birthday. **That coverage effective date (as with all Medicare-related coverages) will be on the first of the month in question.**

The Medicare Part A cost sharing provisions (the amount of medical expenses you, the insured, will be required to pay) are as follows in 2019:

Medicare Part A hospital deductible	$1,364
1st – 60th day inpatient (you pay per day)	$ 0
61st – 90th day coinsurance (you pay)	$ 341
91st – 150th day coinsurance (you pay)	$ 682
151st day on – you pay (no upper limit)	100%

Skilled nursing facility	
First 20 days you pay	$ 0
Days 21 – 100 you pay (per day)	$170.50
Days 101 on you pay (no upper limit)	100%

Generally, someone turning 65 may enroll up to three months before the birthday month begins. Coverage will then go into effect on the 1st day of that birthday month. They also have a few months available to enroll after the birth month, but this might mean going without coverage for some period.

- Exception: if the actual date of birth is on the 1st of any month, coverages will become effective on the 1st day of the prior month.

  Don't ask why this is so; nobody knows.

- Exception: if the existing health insurance plan is an HSA (Health Savings Account) and you would like to continue making pre-tax contributions, it might be wise to consult an expert about delaying enrollment as coverage by Part A may preclude deductible HSA plan contributions.

ENROLL IN MEDICARE PART A ONLINE HERE:

https://www.ssa.gov/medicare/

The enrollment process may possibly take as few as 10 minutes.

CHAPTER 4
Medicare Part B

At the risk of belaboring the obvious, the following is my official definition of the second part of Medicare.

MEDICARE PART B is health insurance provided by the Federal government. It is generally intended to reimburse some expenses incurred during treatment by doctors, testing & diagnostics, medical equipment, supplies and preventive care.

It is very important to choose the effective date of your Part B coverage carefully. Medicare Part B carries a substantial monthly premium (starting at $135.50/month in 2019) so it would not be prudent to start it too early.

More importantly, since Medicare Part B is critically important protection designed to reimburse the costs of the most commonly encountered treatment, it would REALLY not be prudent to enroll too late.

Medicare Part B cost sharing provisions (the amounts you, the insured, are required to pay) are as follows in 2019:

Medicare Part B calendar year deductible$ 185.00

Medicare Part B coinsurance (you pay – no limit)   20%

Late enrollment for Part B, after becoming eligible, risks incurring hefty medical expenses without insurance protection.

If one fails to enroll until after the eligibility period, the opportunity to enroll will be limited to a short period at the beginning of each following year and coverage will not become effective for several months after that.

In addition, substantially late enrollment in Part B subjects one to a lifetime monetary penalty that will be added to the monthly premium forever.

The importance of timely Part B enrollment cannot be stated too strongly.

Turning age 65:

Medicare eligible people who are responsible for their own health insurance will have no difficulty choosing an enrollment date. They will turn age 65 and will properly enroll with an effective date of the first day of their 65th birth month.

- Exception: if the actual date of birth is on the 1st of any month, coverage will become effective on the 1st day of the **prior** month.

    Don't ask why this is so; nobody knows.

The enrollment period begins 3 months before the birth month, and prudence dictates that the enrollment process should begin as early as practical within that 90-day period.

Retirement from a group medical plan after turning 65:

Medicare coverages should be scheduled to begin when the group plan terminates.

It is not prudent to have any gap in coverage and it is really bad to have a gap lasting longer than 63 continuous days. At that point your medical history might come into play as to when you will be allowed to have full coverage for all medical conditions.

Other circumstances that might affect your coverage decisions:

- Do you have a spouse who is actively employed?
- Are you not a US citizen?

- Are you on COBRA or retiree medical coverage from an employer?
- Are you covered by Tricare?
- Do you fall into another category that complicates things?

If any of the above apply, you may need professional advice about whether, or exactly when to begin Medicare Part B coverage. You should seek that advice from any of the unbiased sources I have listed **below.**

ENROLL IN MEDICARE PART B ONLINE HERE:
https://www.ssa.gov/medicare/

The enrollment process may take as few as 10 minutes.

Some unbiased sources of information and advice on choosing the proper Medicare effective date for you:

www.Medicare.gov

https://www.ssa.gov/medicare/
SSA: The Social Security Administration

Choosing a Medigap Policy: A Guide to Health Insurance for People with Medicare:

https://www.medicare.gov/Pubs/pdf/02110-Medicare-Medigap.guide.pdf?

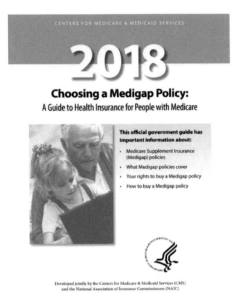

Public service agencies, like a local hospital for instance, may have a Medicare and Social Security advisor on staff.

Your company HR department

Medicare & You 2019:

file:///C:/Users/User/Documents/1%20MIS/BOOK/2019/10050-Medicare-and-You.pdf

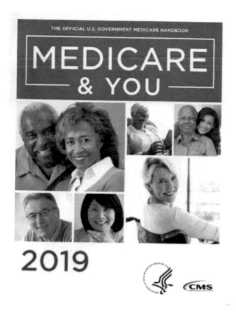

Medicare for Dummies Cheat Sheet

http://www.dummies.com/personal-finance/insurance/health-insurance/medicare-for-dummies-cheat-sheet/

CHAPTER 5

Medicare Is Not Enough Protection!

If you have started the Medicare enrollment process with plenty of time to spare before the effective or starting date, of your coverage, take a break. Do something more fun or productive until your Medicare ID card arrives.

Eventually, you will receive the new Medicare ID card in the mail. It will show your unique alpha/numeric "identifier" and the start dates for Parts A and B.

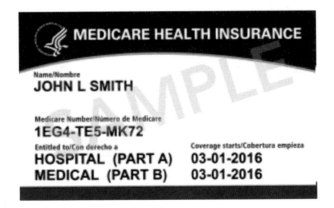

Now is the time to purchase the insurance that will protect you from the dangerous gaping holes in Medicare protection.

What are these gaping holes you ask? They are the deductibles, coinsurance, co-pays and unlimited lifetime cost sharing amounts that severely limit the protection afforded by original Medicare.

These cost sharing elements of Medicare Part A and Part B have no statutory limit. Potentially, very large amounts of money are at risk for people on Medicare who have not purchased additional protection from a private insurance company.

Insurance to supplement Medicare

Two basic types of insurance are available to protect you from financial disaster but only one is worthwhile –

a. **MEDICARE SUPPLEMENT PLANS** – The best and only choice for health insurance to supplement Medicare, assuming you can afford a modest monthly premium cost.

Medicare supplement plans cover the range from very inexpensive and cost-effective HDF – High Deductible Plan F - to the highly popular and benefit rich Plan F, which usually has a pretty darn reasonable cost.

MEDICARE SUPPLEMENTS GIVE YOU FREEDOM!

Read the next two chapters (6 & 7) to learn why I only recommend Medicare supplements to all of my clients.

    b. **MEDICARE ADVANTAGE PLANS (PART C)** – Do not even consider these or waste your time learning about them.

The only reason you hear about Medicare Advantage plans so often is that they pay very generous commissions to the insurance agent – thanks in large part to you, the American taxpayer.

You can read more about Medicare Advantage (Part C) plans in **Chapter 8** if you want to kill some time.

CHAPTER 6

Medicare Supplement Plans– The ONLY Way to Fly!

When compared with the highly-flawed Medicare Advantage (Part C) plans, Medicare supplement plans have only one disadvantage: they are not given away free of charge.

Each Medicare supplement plan has a monthly premium charge, although the costs vary widely between insurance carriers and type of plan.

The available plans are standardized from company to company and each is denoted by a letter. So, as an example, Plan A provides the same protections and benefits no matter which company sells it.

There are eleven Medicare Supplement plans being sold to Medicare eligibles and they all have one great thing in common:

COMPLETE FREEDOM OF CHOICE!

1) Medicare supplement plans never have restrictive networks of doctors and hospitals. A person covered by a Medicare supplement plan is free to seek treatment from any provider who accepts Medicare patients.

2) No network means no lists to consult when it comes to figuring out what providers to use, no risk of nasty surprises when seeking treatment away from home or in an emergency situation.

3) A patient covered by a Medicare supplement may seek treatment from any specialist anywhere without requesting permission from a gate-keeper.

4) Medicare supplement plans, just like Medicare Parts A & B, are good anywhere in the 50 US states and possessions. The two plans I recommend also have a $50,000 lifetime benefit for emergency treatment in foreign countries.

5) A cautionary note: After the initial period of eligibility, insurance companies may question your medical history if you apply for a different plan or to a different company. My advice is to choose your carrier and your supplement plan very carefully because you just may have that plan for the rest of your life.

How does one decide which of the eleven Medicare supplement plans to purchase?

Follow my recommendation to buy either the luxurious Cadillac or the high-performance Pontiac GTO of Medicare supplement plans.

LOTS OF BANG FOR A REASONABLE AMOUNT OF BUCKS!

Two Medicare supplement plans I recommend for the average consumer:

The most comprehensive coverage allowed by law:
PLAN F – the luxurious Cadillac!

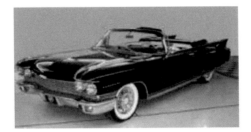

-OR -

Great protection at an exceedingly low price:
HIGH DEDUCTIBLE PLAN F – the high-performance Pontiac GTO!

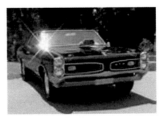

Each of these Medicare supplement plans pay **100%** of the following costs, filling in the many gaps in original Medicare:

Part A deductible
Part A coinsurance and hospital costs
(up to an additional 365 days after Medicare benefits are exhausted)
Part A hospice care coinsurance or copayment

Part B deductible
Part B coinsurance or copayment
Part B excess charges

Skilled nursing facility care coinsurance

Blood (first 3 pints)

AND:
80% of foreign travel emergency expenses after a small deductible
(up to a $50,000 lifetime total)

As you might have guessed, **PLAN F** has no deductibles, co-pays, co-insurance nor any other cost sharing provisions. The insured person will not receive any invoices for routine cost sharing expenses.

As you might also have guessed, **HIGH DEDUCTIBLE PLAN F (HDF)** includes a front-end deductible in exchange for a greatly reduced monthly premium cost. The insured person will receive occasional invoices for small portions of the cost of medical treatment.

Most frequently, these invoices will be for outpatient expenses normally covered by Medicare Part B. Medicare has an annual $185 deductible (in 2019) and then a 20% coinsurance for Part B treatment costs.

I explain in **Chapter 7** that the term "High Deductible" is a complete misnomer, since Medicare pays benefits no matter what supplement plan – if any – is in place.

CHAPTER 7

HDF - The Best Kept Secret in Medicare!

HIGH DEDUCTIBLE PLAN F is a terrific combination of cost vs. benefits! Too bad most agents won't talk about it.

Instead of paying $158 for the very rich PLAN F, save $110 per month and only pay $48 for HDF (see example below). The name "high deductible" is completely misleading and the downside risk is much less than they would have you believe!

As stated elsewhere, this book is written with a particular audience in mind: those who are not infirm and those who are not destitute.

This group can generally afford to pay the reasonable price of regular PLAN F, the Cadillac and most popular of Medicare supplement plans.

However, as rich as are the benefits of PLAN F, it may not be the smartest purchase for most.

My healthy clients always appreciate the cost/benefit of HDF once it is properly explained to them that the term "HIGH DEDUCTIBLE" is a complete misnomer.

The often-overlooked fact is that **MEDICARE PAYS ITS BENEFITS FIRST**, without regard to what kind of supplemental coverage is in place.

This means Medicare pays 100% of **hospital costs** (to a limit) after a reasonable deductible and 80% coverage (with no limit) for **outpatient expenses** after a small deductible, even if there is no supplement in place. In the rare event of a disastrous series of medical expenses, the downside risk of HDF is very reasonable indeed.

Let's look at an example: a client age 65 in Chicago or northern Illinois with Blue Cross/Blue Shield Medicare supplement:

2018 monthly premium for PLAN F	$ 158
2018 monthly premium for HDF	$ 48
Monthly savings	$ 110
Annual savings with HDF	$1,320

In summary, PLAN F pays for everything allowed by law. A holder of PLAN F will not be "balance billed" for any deductibles, co-pays, co-insurance or other costs. Monthly premium in the above example is $158.

HIGH DEDUCTIBLE PLAN F (HDF) covers exactly the same risks, but the insured will have to pay the Medicare Part A deductible ($1,364) and/or the Part B deductible ($185) and/or the Part B coinsurance (20%) until he has paid $2,240 of expenses out of pocket after Medicare pays their share.

After that the coverage under HDF is 100%, just like it is under PLAN F. Monthly premium in the example is $48.

Now, take the potential of paying that $2,240 deductible during a year of unusually high medical expenses, and subtract the annual premium savings of $1,320. The amount at risk is only $920 (about $75 per month) in the absolute worst-case scenario!

With the potential of premium savings in every other year of normal medical expenditures, HIGH DEDUCTIBLE PLAN F is a sure winner for the vast majority of healthy people.

Why, then, is HDF such a well-kept secret?

Low commissions!

Many agents won't discuss this great product without being prodded because it doesn't pay generous commissions.

It would be difficult for an insurance agent to make a living on the paltry commission level paid by companies on such a low-cost product.

Agents earn more when the product they sell is more costly.

If you decide to purchase HDF, bad luck for agents translates to big savings for you!

Try doing the calculations for your own situation and see what you think!

CHAPTER 8

Medicare Advantage (Part C) Plans: Why Not?

The only advantage I can see in Medicare Advantage plans is that they don't cost very much to buy. In fact, many of these plans have $0 monthly premiums! Good deal, right?

Sure, they can be a pretty good deal if nothing bad happens to you; no serious injury or illness that causes the need for medical treatment. In other words, you will be just fine with a Medicare Advantage plan until you actually need to use it.

Insurance agents love these plans because of the generous commissions they pay, thanks to the largess of the taxpayers.

Where are the flaws in Medicare Advantage or Part C plans for the potential customers like you?

NO FREEDOM OF CHOICE!

1) MEDICARE ADVANTAGE (Part C) plans are HMOs or PPOs. They all rely on networks of physicians and hospitals to deliver care. This adds the complication of having to check a list of names to ensure your treatment will be covered.

2) The networks are constantly in flux, with some doctors quitting and others joining. If your favorite doctor were to quit your network, you would be stuck finding a replacement from the list given to you by the insurance company.

3) Costly complications can spring out of the bushes to cause unpleasant surprises. For example, your surgeon might belong to the network but the anesthesiologist he uses may not; the x-ray tech may be in the network but the radiologist may not be. In these examples, you should expect to receive a hefty invoice in the mail.

4) Frequently, permission is required prior to seeking consultation with a specialist.

5) Networks often operate in localized areas and traveling out of them or living in a second

home somewhere can be a problem, if medical treatment is needed.

6) The Medicare advantage plans will promise that out-of-network emergency care is covered, but may balk at cooperating when it comes to actually paying for it.

SOMETIMES WE GET WHAT WE PAY FOR!

Medicare Advantage plans generally have lots of cost sharing: deductibles, co-pays, co-insurance and out-of-pocket costs to the insured exceeding $6,000 per year in many cases.

Few of their customers ask what their plan's annual per person out-of-pocket limit is, which leads to unpleasant surprises when medical expenses are incurred!

Also, the many extras they tout, like dental, hearing and vision coverage are often disappointing limited benefit discount plans rather than true insurance.

How can an insurance company give away a product for free? This only works if the government pays the freight. When the government decides to cut its expenses, the insured clients will be the ones to pick up the slack.

The good news is that holders of Medicare Advantage (Part C) plans are allowed to switch from one plan or company to another every year during AEP or Open Enrollment, which allows dissatisfied subscribers to try out a new plan effective the following January 1st.

Have you noticed that there is a huge amount of direct mail, TV ads, internet pop-ups and other annoying insurance talk happening every fall?
This is because the poor saps who found themselves stuck with Medicare Advantage plans have an opportunity to try something else.... anything else to replace the crapola they bought last year.

Once again, **I do not recommend Medicare Advantage (Part C) plans** for my audience of Medicare eligibles who are not destitute or infirm.

CHAPTER 9

Drugs? We Don't Need No Stinkin' Drugs!

PDP, Prescription Drug Plan or Part D – buy it ASAP!

In their infinite generosity, the Feds now subsidize the cost of prescription drug plans that can be purchased from private insurance companies.

Each of these companies can price their drug plans where they want to, compile their own list of drugs to be covered (formulary) and offer different levels of benefit to their customers.

Here are the problems: the construction of each drug plan sounds very complicated to the non-insurance professional; there are deductibles, co-pays, co-insurance and a big scary donut hole to contend with.

Additionally, the formularies and premiums can change from one year to the next and each individual's prescription medication requirements can change.

Therefore, I recommend comparing all available plans only on the basis of the estimated out of pocket cost per year. If the changes in formulary, premium cost or drug needs warrant, the insured can move to a new company and a new plan during the annual open enrollment.

There is a fairly painless way to compare the cost of all of the drug plans in your locality via the government website and I have easy navigation directions **below.**

What if you are so healthy that you take no prescription drugs at all? After thanking the ancestors who passed down your particular gene pool, consider whether there might be a need for insuring against high prescription costs anytime in the future.

If not, and you expect to never, ever purchase one of these drug plans, you are finished right now.

On the other hand, most people without crystal balls like to keep their options open and hedge their bets. And they generally want to avoid the lifetime late enrollment penalty.

If a person becomes eligible to purchase a PDP but elects not to do that, and then decides to go ahead and buy one sometime in the future, a late enrollment penalty will be assessed for each month elapsed from the initial eligibility period to the actual purchase.

The penalty amounts to roughly 35 cents per month for each month elapsed. That means an extra $4.20 per month for a one-year delay, $8.40 per month for a two-year delay, $12.60 per month for a three-year delay and so on.

This is why I advise my clients to buy an inexpensive PDP (maybe $22 per month) when they are first eligible, even if they take no drugs yet.

Admittedly, not all have followed my advice, but I sleep better at night knowing that I tried.

Kind of like child rearing.

SELECT THE LOWEST COST PDP PLAN

NAVIGATION INSTRUCTIONS
START HERE: WWW.MEDICARE.GOV

1) Go to the site; Click on green button labelled: "FIND HEALTH & DRUG PLANS"

2) Under "Basic Search" enter the appropriate ZIP Code and click "FIND PLANS"

3) Click on three answers:
- "I DON'T KNOW WHAT COVERAGE I HAVE"
- "I DON'T KNOW"
- "YES"

Click brown button "CONTINUE TO PLAN RESULTS"

4) Inside the green box "TYPE THE NAME OF YOUR DRUG"
- In the drop-down box select the dosage, frequency and pharmacy
- Click on brown button "ADD DRUG AND DOSAGE"
- Repeat as needed until all drugs have been entered
- Click brown button "MY DRUG LIST IS COMPLETE"

5) Inside the green box, choose the greatest number of miles available
- Select up to two pharmacies of your choice
- Click brown button "CONTINUE TO PLAN RESULTS"

6) Inside the green box: check the box next to "PRESCRIPTION DRUG PLANS (WITH ORIGINAL MEDICARE)"

Click brown button: "CONTINUE TO PLAN RESULTS"

7) Final page is entitled: "YOUR PLAN RESULTS"
   • Plans listed in order of "Remainder of Year Retail Costs", lowest to highest
   • Plans can be sorted by "Remainder of Year Mail Order Costs", among other criteria

8) Click the box next to the name of the plan of your choice, and then do the same for one or two more likely choices. Then move up the page and click "Compare".

You will be taken to a thorough comparison of the annual costs for both retail and mail order purchase of the drugs on your list, as well as enrollment information for each plan. A star rating of 3 or better is considered acceptable.

Consider repeating this process each year at Annual Enrollment Period (AEP) in the fall.

CHAPTER 10

What Will All of This Cost?

There is a monetary cost for all insurance coverage and government supplied health insurance is no exception. The good news is that, if you are coming off an Obamacare type of plan, the new costs will look like a bargain to you!

A note about IRMAA – the success penalty. This stands for Income Related Monthly Adjustment Amount and adds to the monthly premium based on what the IRS has recorded as your MAGI (Modified Adjusted Gross Income) two years ago.

The target audience for this book is likely to encounter the following monthly premium costs in 2019:

Medicare Part A   Free of Charge

Medicare Part B $135.50
      (IRMAA could increase it substantially)

See full Medicare Part B IRMAA chart **below**.

Medicare Supplement Plans: Premiums vary widely depending on several factors, including state of residence, age, sex, ZIP code and sometimes smoking status

HIGH DEDUCTIBLE PLAN F – most cost effective – estimated between $30 and $80

PLAN F – most comprehensive - estimated between $140 & $250

Prescription Drug Plans (PDP) - $18 and up, depending on plan and location plus drug deductibles, co-pays and co-insurance.

PDPs are also subject to an IRMAA penalty assessment.

See full Prescription Drug Plan (PDP) IRMAA chart **below**.

The **Income Related Monthly Adjustment Amount** charts below are based on Modified Adjusted Gross Income reported to the IRS two years prior.

IRMAA Penalties for
MEDICARE PART B PREMIUMS

IF YOU:

FILE INDIVIDUALLY	FILE JOINTLY	PART B PREMIUM
$85,000 or less	$170,000 or less	$135.50
$85K to $107K	$170K to $214K	$189.60
$107K to $133.5K	$214K to $267K	$270.90
$133.5K to $160K	$267K to $320K	$352.20
$160K to $500K	$320K to $750K	$433.40
$500K or more	$750K or more	$460.50

IRMAA Penalties for
PRESCRIPTION DRUG PLANS

IF YOU:

FILE INDIVIDUALLY	FILE JOINTLY	PDP PREMIUM PLUS
$85,000 or less	$170,000 or less	$0
$85K to $107K	$170K to $214K	$12.40
$107K to $133.5K	$214K to $267K	$31.90
$133.5K to $160K	$267K to $320K	$51.40
$160K to $500K	$320K to $750K	$70.90
$500K or more	$750K or more	$77.40

CHAPTER 11

Did You Make A Boo-Boo?

It is very likely that you are hearing about the excellent benefits of Medicare supplement plans and especially the great cost advantage of HIGH DEDUCTIBLE PLAN F (HDF) for the first time.

Since commissions payable to agents are more substantial for Medicare Advantage plans, those are the ones that are promoted most vigorously to the unsuspecting public.

Is that the case with you?

Were you kept in the dark about Medicare supplements and HDF?

Are you anxious to make a change so that you can enjoy the benefits of Medicare supplement plans along with all of my happy clients?

Well, I have good news and bad news for you:

GOOD NEWS: You may apply for a Medicare supplement policy from an insurance carrier any time the mood strikes!

BAD NEWS: There is no "guaranteed issue" period for Medicare supplement plans after your initial enrollment period when you first became eligible. You MAY be asked a series of questions about your medical history in order to prove that you are insurable.

This is not true in every instance or in every state but generally you will have to jump through some hoops in order to be allowed to buy a Medicare supplement policy outside of the initial enrollment period. You might be refused if your medical condition and history do not meet the insurance company's insurability standards.

There are a few special exceptions but understanding them and the related complexities is what makes Medicare so much fun.

My website (coming soon) may be able to help,
depending on where you live:
www.MedicareInSeconds.com

MEDICARE
IN SECONDS

CONTACT ME:

DBJ@MedicareInSeconds.com

ACKNOWLEDGMENTS

This book would not exist. I would still be sitting at my desk with fingers poised over the keys and eyes caressing the mountains around our Arizona home were it not for my wife.

Mary is among my most rabid critics but can often be brought around to my way of thinking with some persistent persuasion. Once on my team, she is an invaluable asset and a source of insight, inspiration, motivation and support.

Mary is not really high maintenance, but she does need to be reminded periodically that "spousal unit" is actually a term of loving endearment. Not much else to say after almost 50 years of partnership and teamwork.

Thanks to my personal clients who helped me form the idea for this project after realizing why they were all so frustrated.

Others, generally without being pestered, have explained complicated technological mysteries, prodded me out of lethargy or sharpened red pencils to gleefully perform surgery on my sterling prose.

They have shared companionship, cocktails, encouragement, ribald jokes and philosophical pontification, all without ever a negative word about this relatively ambitious project. So I also thank, in no particular order:

Randy & Margaret Carson of C2C Consulting, LLC
Brian and Teri Jones
Paul and Kathleen Bowling
Gerry and Lisa Schafer
Roy and Kathy Brotherhood
Tony and Melisa Coletto

Finally, for no reason other than I just enjoy them, I must acknowledge the youngest generation of my gene pool. Thanks for making the rest of us proud and happy to have you in our family:

Max Coletto & Alex Coletto - Californians just starting to spread their wings.

Drew McMillin, Robbie McMillin and Kate McMillin – Canadian-Americans proud to wave both flags.

Made in the
USA
Middletown, DE